Moringa Oleifera

The Tree of Life

"And the leaves of the tree were for the healing of the nations." Rev. 22:2c

Dexter & Petula Jones

Uwriteitpublishing Company
Goldsboro, NC 27534

*Moringa Oleifera-The Tree of Life by Dexter &
Petula Jones*
Copyright © 2018 Dexter & Petula Jones

ISBN-13: 978-1729875193
ISBN-10: 172987519X

First Printing—December 2018

This publication is designed to provide information in
regard to the subject matter covered. It is published with
the understanding that the author is not engaged in
rendering legal counsel or other professional services. It is
for educational purposes only. If legal advice or other
professional advice is required, the services of a
professional person should be sought.

- These statements have not been evaluated by the
  Food & Drug Administration. This product
  information is not intended to diagnose, treat,
  cure or prevent any diseases.
- Scripture quotations are from the King James
  Version of the Bible unless otherwise stated.

"Let Moringa be your medicine and your medicine be Moringa."

"And by the river upon the bank thereof, on this side and on that side, shall grow all trees for meat, whose leaf shall not fade, neither shall the fruit thereof be consumed: it shall bring forth new fruit according to his months, because their waters they issued out of the sanctuary: and the fruit thereof shall be for meat, **and the leaf thereof for medicine.."** *Ezekiel 47:12*

"A New You Today, The Moringa Way."

"He causeth the grass to grow for the cattle, and herb for the service (the aid, assistance and help) of man: that he may bring forth food out of the earth." Psalms 104:14

"Moringa is the most powerful superfood ever discovered by mankind. It's the only plant that supplies our bodies with all the essential nutrients needed for a healthy body in one single plant."

"And out of the ground made the LORD God to grow every tree that is pleasant to the sight, and good for food; the tree of life also in the midst of the garden, and the tree of knowledge of good and evil."
Genesis 2:9

"Moringa Oleifera is often called "The Miracle Tree" because of the enormous health benefits that one derives from using it."

Table of Contents

Acknowledgements
About the Authors
Foreword

Acknowledgements

I would like to first off acknowledge the Creator and Maker of all plant life and human life—God Almighty. Whatever mankind thinks he has discovered he has only brought to the surface God's creation and therefore the honor and glory belongs to God Almighty. Moringa Oleifera is God's plant and we're privileged to be able to distribute and sell it to help individuals to meet their health and wellness needs and to get their health back. We acknowledge all our customers that has patronize our business in the past and that will patronize it in the future. God bless you all.

About the Authors

Dexter & Petula Jones is first and foremost Ministers of the gospel of Jesus Christ. Evangelists, that believes in going beyond the church walls to reach the lost with the good news of the gospel. Ministry is their first love because God saved them both out of a world of sin and transformed their lives and made them righteous through Jesus Christ. Now they're going about their Father's business letting the world know that Jesus is the Savior of the world and he came to reconcile man back to God.

Their second love is spreading the good news about God's Superfood Moringa Oleifera. This amazing product has changed their life physically and has enabled them to live a healthy life as well as a life of prevention from sickness and diseases. They know firsthand that the goal is wellness and prevention of disease rather than restoring health to a sick body.

The testimonies that they've seen from

Individuals that have used Moringa Oleifera on a consistent basis are in many instances amazing.

The manner in which God brought his creation into their hands is also amazing. In August of 2016 a friend of Dexter's nephew Jomo Jones whose name is Kelo was in town coming from Charlotte and he brought some Moringa back in town with him. He introduced all of us to the product and made us a bottle of Moringa water. He was very positive about the benefits of the product and what it had done for him and many other individuals whose testimonies he heard. So he gave us a bottle of Moringa water and after drinking it the product gave me instant energy. My response was, **"what is in this stuff?"** Kelo gave us each a sample to take home to continue to try it in order to reap all the benefits of this amazing plant.

As a God gifted researcher I begin to delve into the history of **"Moringa Oleifera"** and the more I researched the more amazed I became. Day by day I was learning new information about a product that I had never heard of before. I became obsessed with learning about this product that had changed the life of so many people. The more I learned the more I wanted to learn because I could not believe that one product could do all this. I have studied many herbs for 30 + years but nothing had even come close to Moringa Oleifera in a single plant.

Other herbs it was necessary in many instances to add many herbs together to get the full effect, Moringa Oleifera however was able to stand alone and yet supply the body with all the essential nutrients. This plant was truly amazing and the more I researched the deeper it got as I learned that over 1300 articles have been written about Moringa Oleifera as well as many books about the veracity of this superfood.

My ultimate conclusion was this is too good to keep to myself. I have to let the world (or at least my world and as my as I could reach) know about this plant that can do so many things but has been hidden for many years. I told my wife that this was more than just a great product that came into our hands; we have to get the word out. So after going through different processes of selling and distributing Moringa Oleifera we decided to make it a real business and formulate all the legalities we needed to establish our own health store called **"Eden Wellness Moringa."**

We named it this because we believe that such a tree must have been in the **"Garden of Eden"** when God created his world and placed the man whom he formed. As the scripture states, *"And the LORD God formed man of the dust of the ground, and breathed into his nostrils the breath of life: and man became a living soul. And the LORD God planted a garden eastward in Eden; and there he put the man whom he had formed. And out of the ground made the LORD God to grow every tree (**the Moringa Tree**) that is pleasant to the sight, and good for food; the tree of life also in the midst of the garden, and the tree of the knowledge of good and evil. And a river went* *out of Eden to water the garden."* Genesis 2:7-10a This was the beginning of both Ministry and Business for us to introduce Moringa Oleifera to the world.

FOREWORD

Moringa Oleifera-The Tree of Life is a book that will reveal to the reader about our modern day leaves for the healing of the nation and man's need to get back to the *"herb of the field." Genesis 3:18b* We have become a nation that is consumed with medicine and we're not the better for it. We're more doped up than ever before in spite of our advance in technology and the fact that mankind is smarter than ever.

God never intended for your body to be serviced through medicine but by the herbs of the field. He has created a leaf or a plant for every illness known to man.

In this book we will delve into the most powerful tree ever discovered and reveal what's within the leaves of the Moringa Oleifera tree. The scripture says, *"And the leaves of the tree were for the healing of the nations." Revelation 22:2c* Well it's time for the nations to be healed the way God intended them to be healed and this book will open your eyes from a spiritual as well as a natural perspective. You will learn things about the Garden of Eden and why Adam had to eat of the trees of the garden for sustainability so that his body would be recharged, restored, strengthen, freshen, nourished and empowered.

You will also see how in the New Jerusalem a time will come when the nations or the redeemed shall be gathered out of every nation according to Revelation 21:24 which states *"And the nations of them which are saved shall walk in the light of it: and the kings of the earth do bring their glory and honour into it."* Also the book of Ezekiel 47:12 tells us about the leaves of a tree which will be used for healing as it states, *"And by the river upon the bank thereof, on this side and on that side, shall grow all trees for meat, whose leaf shall not fade, neither shall the fruit thereof be consumed: it shall bring forth new fruit according to his months, because their waters they issued out of the sanctuary: and the fruit thereof shall be for meat, and **the leaf thereof for medicine."***

The nations that do bring their glory in the new Jerusalem will have access to this tree and will need it not to abstain from sickness or disease but to keep their body in health just as Adam had to eat to keep his body in health. You will learn how the leaves of the tree for the healing of the nations are twofold and consist of a future use as well as a present use in our day. Get ready for a revealing of the most powerful leaves ever discovered by mankind—Moringa Oliefera. Here we're not stating that Moringa Oleifera was the tree of life in the Garden of Eden, no, but we're saying as many has already stated that this tree is the modern day tree of life that can restore the body of man back to a place of health and wellness.

"There is a tree that's more amazing than you will ever know and it's a miracle tree that can change your life."

"Now unto him that is able to do exceeding abundantly, above anything you can ask or think."

"Wouldn't it be great to have a tree that could cause your body to repair itself?"

1

The Garden of Eden

"And the LORD God planted a garden eastward in Eden; and there he put the man whom he had formed." Genesis 2:8

The word of God tells us about what happened in the beginning of time. Man may have his interpretations or his belief about how the world was formed, but our belief is that *"In the beginning God created the heaven and the earth."* Genesis 1:1

Not only did he create the heavens and the earth but he also created all the animals of the field as well as all trees and vegetation's. The word of God says, *"And God said, Let the earth bring forth grass, the herb yielding seed, and the fruit tree yielding fruit after his kind, whose seed is in itself, upon the earth: and it was so.*

12 And the earth brought forth grass, and herb yielding seed after his kind, and the tree yielding fruit, whose seed was in itself, after his kind: and God saw that it was good.

13 And the evening and the morning were the third day. "Genesis 1:11-13

Within this garden God had called forth all manner of trees that would be good for food for the man that he was about to put in the garden. This type of garden made by God was indeed the garden of gardens. The word Eden means **"Paradise"** or a place of luxurious living; it was indeed a place of pleasure. Within this garden was everything that man could desire for his spiritual life and his physical life. Spiritually, God would come and commune with him in the cool of the day. Physically, God had brought for the trees that would be for his nutrition.

The Garden of Eden was a place of happiness and peace. Man had everything that his heart could desire, he was in charge of all the animals and everything was obedient to his command.

He also had every plant, herb and tree that was essential for helping to sustain his physical body because at this time he did not have eternal life in him. *"5 And every plant of the field before it was in the earth, and every herb of the field before it grew: for the LORD God had not caused it to rain upon the earth, and there was not a man to till the ground.*

6 But there went up a mist from the earth, and watered the whole face of the ground." Genesis 2:5-6

Among the trees of the Garden we are of the belief that the Moringa Oleifera tree was there also. This belief is backed up with the word of God that states *"And out of the ground made the LORD God to grow **every tree** that is pleasant to the sight, **and good for food;** the tree of life also in the midst of the garden, and the tree of knowledge of good and evil."* Genesis 2:9

The Moringa Oleifera tree was somewhere within the garden and man had access to this amazing tree and could freely eat of it. The trees of the garden at that time were true Superfoods that were created for a Superman called Adam. This man was God's most prized possession and nothing was too good for him. Every tree within this garden was his for food except the tree of the knowledge of good and evil.

We can't even begin to fathom the body of Adam and how lively it was before the fall. But just to give you an earthly perspective of what his body must have been like and this in no way does it justice. But Adam's body was:

- Full of life

- Vibrant

- Dynamic

- Healthy

- Flourishing

- Thriving

- Totally Alive

- Robust

- Nothing Missing

- Nothing Lacking

- Whole

- Top Form

- Full of Strength

- Sound

What Adam possesses physically was out of this world but his body still did not possess eternal life within it. In order for Adam's body to possess eternal life he would have had to eat of the tree of life that was in the midst of the garden. Do you see here how everything that deals with Adam relates to trees? This is why God gave the command to the Angels after the fall to get them out of the garden lest they eat of the tree of life and live forever in their sinful state. The word of God says, "*And the LORD God said, Behold, the man is become as one of us, to know good and evil: and now, **lest he put forth his hand, and take also of the tree of life, and eat, and live for ever:** Therefore the LORD God sent him forth from the garden of Eden, to till the ground from whence he was taken.*" Genesis 3:22-23

Adam never ate of the tree of life so that his body could possess eternal life so therefore his body succumb to weakness after he ate of the forbidden tree. God wanted man to live forever and before he was able to eat of the tree of life he was given a probationary period to live and his physical body was daily replenished as he ate of the trees that were *good for food in the garden.*

When he ate of these trees his body was recharged, restored, freshen, nourished and empowered. The trees of the garden were for this specific purpose.

The scriptures does not tell us exactly how long Adam lived before he was exiled out of the garden but during that time he had to eat and the trees were his meat or food.

Every tree of the garden was provided for his physical pleasure and he had a variety to choose from. There were such trees as:

1. Fruit trees

2. Avocado trees

3. Fig trees

4. Nut trees

5. Trees with leaves for food

6. And many others…

The fact that God gave them food to eat suggests that their bodies were designed to eat and digest food for the sustaining of their physical body. Eating was a privilege that was permitted by God and he knew they would eat and would enjoy eating. His only requirement was that they could not eat of just one tree in the garden and that was the tree of the knowledge of good and evil. The eating of this tree would cause immediate spiritual death which would result in eventual physical death of their bodies.

Their bodies just as ours needed essential nutrients to sustain it and God gave them the nutrients in the food and leaves of the trees. Without eating the essential nutrients daily their bodies would have become malnutrition and eventual physical death would occur but God knew physical death would never occur from this perspective because eating was a pleasure which they would always enjoy.

Right now if you're sick in any form or fashion your body is craving for the 90+ essential nutrients that it needs for satisfaction. Your body wants to get back as close as possible to the feeling of liveliness it felt in the Garden of Eden. It will never get back 100% but it groans to live once again with the feeling of vibrancy. We cannot return to the Garden of Eden but God has not left mankind without a remedy that's capable of sustaining his physical body as much as possible until the time comes *when this corruption shall put on incorruption and this mortal shall put on immortality. 1 Corinthians 15:*

2

The Tree of Life

"Let Moringa be thy medicine and thy medicine be Moringa."

Because of the disobedience and sin of Adam mankind was plunged into darkness and his spirit and physical body suffers today as a result of this darkness. Adam's once lively body begin to deteriorate and weaken until finally it died and returned to the dust of the ground. It took Adam over 900 years to die physically because his physical body was permeating with the life of God and it had to learn how to die through deterioration. *"And all the days that Adam lived were nine hundred and thirty years and he died."* *Genesis 5:5* The body of Adam begin the process of becoming progressively worse. His health begin to decline, fail, collapse, drop and go on a downward slump until it had no more life in it. His once vibrant body began to descend from a higher level pulsating with life to a lower level of feebleness and eventually death.

Mankind has gone physically from been able to live to a ripe old age of 969 years old (Methuselah) to an age of merely 70 years if he's fortunate enough to live this long. His body has unfortunately deteriorated to the point that at times he/she only lives a few years in the case of children dying with diseases ravaging their bodies.

Mankind in this life will never see the days of 900 years ever again on this side of life, only during the 1000 year reign of Christ and when the new heaven and new earth is established. Nevertheless, we still need to take care of our temple which is our body to the best of our abilities. We need to take better care in the form of dietary, exercise and supplying our body with what it's deficient in on a daily basis.

Daily, you have all kinds of diseases and sicknesses that's pulling on your body and trying to invade your cells and enter your bloodstream to make you sick. Many times your body will fight off these things because God has created it to resist many foreign enemies that shouldn't enter it. However, when your body is deficient in the essential vitamins and minerals that's there to assist you these enemies will have a loophole and enter through an opening that's unprotected and lack resistance.

Many essential vitamins and minerals are there to aid, help and assist our bodies in the fight to protect us but when they're lacking the door is opened and sickness is the inevitable end result. God never originally intended for your body to deal with sickness and disease, it was never a part of God's original purpose. God always had high thoughts for mankind and his will is that mankind will be whole in spirit, soul and body. To be whole in spirit yet deficient in soul is still a life out of balance. To be whole in spirit and soul yet deficient in body still isn't God's best for mankind. The word of God says, *"Beloved, I wish above all things that thou mayest prosper and be in health, even as thy soul prospereth."* 3 John 2

If your body is currently experiencing any type of disease (dis-ease), illness, sickness, discomfort, ailment, complication, disorder, bug, infirmity, malady, trouble, infection, contagion, attack, bout, fit, feebleness, debility, weakness, frailness, lameness, malady, unsoundness, distemper, epidemic, pest, plague, agitation, disturbance, distress, irritation, etc… then you are not walking in perfect health even though you are fearfully and wonderfully made. Sickness and disease is not what your body was created for, it's an enemy of your body. Your body was created by your Creator to be healthy and never get sick.

- Sickness is an invasion.

- Sickness is an adversary.

- Sickness is an enemy.

- Sickness is a foreigner.

- Sickness is a negative.

- Sickness is a foe.

- Sickness is an opponent.

- Disease is rivalry.

- Disease is nemesis.

- Disease is a curse.

- Disease is an affliction.

- Disease is a minus.

- Disease is a liability.

- Disease is of the devil.

You are fearfully and wonderfully made

by your Creator to be full of life with the absent of sickness. However, sickness will not just stay off your body because you want it to, you must do the things necessary not to get sick.

There is only one tree that has been called **the tree of life** today that can supply your body with all the essential nutrients needed in one tree. That tree is called Moringa Oleifera. You may ask what makes this a tree of life. Well, when God created the Moringa Oleifera tree he placed within that tree all the nutrients that our body need in a single tree. There is no other tree on the planet that can be given that right but Moringa Oleifera. It's amazing the nutrients that it contains, Moringa has:

- **3 times the Potassium in bananas.**

- **7 times the Vitamin-C as in oranges.**

- **25 times the Iron in spinach.**

- 4 times the Calcium in milk.

- 4 times the Vitamin A in Carrots.

- 46 + Antioxidants

- 36 Anti-Inflammatory Compounds

- 90 + Nutrients

- 18 + Amino Acids

- 8 Essential Amino Acids—the one your body cannot survive without but cannot manufacture on its own.

- 20 times more Vitamin E than Tofu.

- 2 times more Protein than Eggs.

- 10 times more Vitamin E than Nuts.

- Moringa contains Omega-3, 6, & 9.

- Vitamins: A, B1, B2, B3, B5, B6, B7,

B8, B9 B12, C, D, E, K, Choline, Flavonoids.

- **Minerals:** Calcium, Magnesium, Phosphorus, Potassium, Sodium, Sulfur, Cobalt, Copper, Aluminum, Arsenic, Barium, Beryllium, Boron, Bromine, Carbon, Iodine, Iron, Manganese, Selenium, Zinc, Cerium, Cesium, Chromium, Dysprosium, Erbium, Europium, Gadolinium, Gallium, Germanium, Gold, Hafnium, Holmium, Hydrogen, Lanthanum, Lithium, Lutetium, Molybdenum, Neodymium, Nickel, Niobium, Nitrogen, Oxygen, Praseodymium, Rhenium, Rubidium, Samarium, Scandium, Silica, Silver, Strontium, Tantalum, Terbium, Thulium, Tin, Titanium, Vanadium, Ytterbium, Yttrium, Zirconium. **All in 1 tree**

There is no other tree on the planet that can give your body all these nutrients in 1 single tree.

Many times we experience various sickness and diseases because we are deficient in vitamins and minerals. When you're lacking essential nutrients then your body begins to work against you instead of with you.

There are divine miracles where God supernaturally heals your body through the gifts of the spirit of healing and miracles. But if you haven't been healed by God's miraculous power there is no reason for you to remain sick. God in his wisdom have created a miracle tree whose leaves can cause your body to repair itself. This is no ordinary tree and it cannot be grouped with all the other trees in the world. This tree is extraordinary and with all the nutrients in Moringa it has been discovered that this amazing plant has the highest protein ratio of any plant analyzed so far. With such inherited protein it's an absolute that your body will not only survive but thrive as every cell in your body is impacted with the highest protein available today in plant form. Because our bodies use protein to repair and build tissue Moringa is an important building block of our body functions. With such an infusion of essential proteins your body will take care of itself as Moringa both prevent the occurrence of disease as well as slow down the rate or frequency of disease.

Moringa is a product when used on a consistent basis has the power to intervene and deter any evidence of disease or sickness. It has the ability to eliminate problems at the source, thereby preventing the occurrence of an issue. Moringa's aim is to empower your body to be able to sustain itself and thereby reduce the risk of developing diseases.

Moringa Oleifera can aid and assist you to return your body to a normal or healthy condition as God designed it to do. Moringa gets to the source of the problem and helps your body to heal itself as the missing nutrients helps your body to fight off toxins that make it sick while at the same time strengthening your body functions by giving it new life as you absorb the miracle working power of Moringa.

There are several ways Moringa does this to help restore health and wellness to your body.

1. *It detoxifies your body.*

2. *It removes the parasites out of your body.*

3. *It builds up your immune system.*

4. *It fights off free radicals with its rich amount of antioxidants.*

5. *It reduces inflammation in the body.*

6. *It protects the cardiovascular system.*

7. *It helps to support the brain health.*

8. *It helps to protect the liver.*

9. *It helps to protect the kidneys.*

10. *Moringa contains antimicrobial and antibacterial properties.*

11. *Moringa helps to reduce stress.*

12. *It helps to support a healthy digestive system.*

13. *It helps to maintain strong and healthy bones.*

14. *Moringa helps to balance your hormones.*

15. *Moringa protects and nourishes the skin.*

16. *Moringa contains 90+ nutrients to meet your physical needs.*

17. *Moringa contains 36 anti-inflammatory compounds.*

18. *Moringa contains 46 antioxidants.*

19. *Moringa contains 8 essential amino acids which your body needs but cannot produce.*

20. *Moringa contains phytonutrients like*

zeatin, quercetin, beta-sistosterol, caffeeoylquinic acid and kaempferol.

21. Moringa boosts energy level naturally.

Moringa is known by over 100 names in various parts of the world and is now becoming very popular in the United States. In 2008, the National Institute of Health called Moringa Oleifera the **"plant of the year."** Also, according to the ORAC, Moringa scored 157,000, topping all the other antioxidants superfoods on the market today. Including such superfoods as Acai Berries, Green tea, Blueberries, Dark Chocolate, Garlic, Spirulina, Matcha, Turmeric, Etc...

There is no better and more qualified tree today for Prevention or Restoring your health back to normal. Prevention is the key and Restoration is both a process and a journey and Moringa Oleifera is God's modern day Tree of Life that will bring life back into your body.

3

God's Superfood

"The only tree that's truly qualified to be called God's Superfood is Moringa Oleifera."

In order for a plant or tree to be called God's Superfood it must be of superior quality and at the top of the list. Such a product with God's name in the front of it must far exceed anything else on the market today. Such a product must not only have a natural preeminence but will also have a spiritual preeminence.

God's Superfood Moringa Oleifera was one of the trees in the Garden of Eden because this tree was and still is today *"good for food."* Genesis 2:9 Moringa Oleifera is actually a food and not a vitamin or supplement but a food that contains all the vitamins and minerals needed for human consumption. Moringa Oleifera from a spiritual standpoint is absolutely amazing as a food because it has a spiritual effect on your body and mind thereby revitalizing your whole being. As Hippocrates stated many years ago "Let your food be your medicine and your medicine be your food." When Adam ate food his body was able to restore the nutrients that it used up on a daily basis and his body never became depleted or deficient of proper nutrients.

When you're eating the right foods they give your body the proper nutrients to provide it great health, energy and true vitality. When Adam ate of the fruit or leaves of the trees it would strengthen and revitalize his organs. These nutrients provided substance that in turn provided energy for the functions of his body. These nutrients also allowed his body to repair itself and also kept his immune system strong.

If Adam needed food for strength and vitality for his body how much more do we need it for our bodies that are perishing daily. *"Though our outward man perish, yet the inward man is renewed day by day."* 2 *Corinthians 4:16* That's why it's vital that with all our eating we must make sure to include God's Superfood Moringa Oliefera in our daily consumption in one form or another. Food is very important because the body needs a variety of 5 different nutrients and our foods are designed to provide these nutrients. The foods that Adam ate provided his body these 5 essential nutrients.

1. **Proteins**

2. **Carbohydrates**

3. **Fat**

4. **Vitamins**

5. **Minerals**

Moringa Oleifera is the only tree on the planet that provides your body with all 5 nutrients completely in one single plant. This tree is so amazing that without it your body will have to consume a variety of things just to meet the daily need of this one tree. Moringa is a powerhouse of nutrients and it will supercharge your body like nothing else will. The benefits of consuming Moringa daily are staggering and almost unbelievable. Here are the benefits that are derived from this miracle tree.

Information content starting from page (48-72) was contributed by Sandra Toliver. Her body of knowledge about Moringa Oleifera and nutrients are amazing and I'm honored for her contribution in this book.

Moringa Nutritional Benefits-Healthiest Plant on Earth-A Complete Food-All Natural Raw Food

MORINGA'S BENEFITS: are derived from the plant's high concentration of bio-available nutrients. It contains high levels of Vitamin A (beta carotene),

Vitamin B1 (Thiamine), Vitamin B2 (Riboflavin), Vitamin B3 (Niacin), Vitamin B6 (Pyridoxine), Vitamin B7 (Biotin), Vitamin B12 (methylcobalamin), Vitamin C (Ascorbic Acid), Vitamin D (Cholecalciferol), Vitamin E (Tocopherol) and Vitamin K.

Vitamin A (beta carotene) is needed by the retina of the eye in the form of a specific metabolite, the light-absorbing molecule retinal. This molecule is absolutely necessary for both scotopic vision and color vision. Vitamin A also functions in a very different role - as an irreversibly oxidized form retinoic acid, which is an important hormone-like growth factor for epithelial and other cells.

Vitamin B1 (thiamine) helps fuel the body by converting blood sugar into energy. It keeps the mucous membranes healthy and is essential for the nervous system and cardiovascular and muscular functions.

Vitamin B2 (riboflavin) is required for a wide variety of cellular processes. Like the other B vitamins, it plays a key role in energy metabolism, and for the metabolism of fats, ketone bodies, carbohydrates, and proteins. It is the central component of the cofactors FAD and FMN, and is therefore required by all "Flavoproteins".

Vitamin B3 (niacin), like all B complex vitamins, is necessary for healthy skin, hair, eyes, and liver. It also helps the nervous system function properly. Niacin helps the body produce sex and stressrelated hormones in the adrenal glands and other parts of the body. It is effective in improving circulation and reducing cholesterol levels in the blood.

Vitamin B6 (pyridoxine) is required for the synthesis of the neurotransmitters serotonin and norepinephrine and for myelin formation. Pyridoxine deficiency in adults principally affects the peripheral nerves, skin, mucous membranes, and the blood cell system. In children, the central nervous system (CNS) is also affected. Deficiency can occur in people with uremia, alcoholism, cirrhosis, hyperthyroidism, malabsorption syndromes, congestive heart failure (CHF), and in those taking certain medications.

Vitamin B7 (biotin) has vital metabolic functions. Without biotin as a co-factor, many enzymes do not work properly, and serious complications can occur, including varied diseases of the skin, intestinal tract, and nervous system. Biotin can help address high blood glucose levels in people with type 2 diabetes, and is helpful in maintaining healthy hair and nails, decreasing insulin resistance and improving glucose tolerance, and possibly preventing birth defects. It plays a role in energy metabolism, and has been used to treat alopecia, cancer, Crohn's disease, hair loss, Parkinson's disease, peripheral neuropathy, Rett syndrome, seborrheic dermatitis, and vaginal candidiasis.

Vitamin B12 (Inserted by Dexter L. Jones) (Methylcobalamin) Methylcobalamin is the specific form of B12 needed for nervous system health. Vitamin B12 plays an important role in helping the body make red blood cells. Methylcobalamin is a water-soluble vitamin. The body uses vitamin B12 in energy production and regulation, among other metabolic roles.

Vitamin C (ascorbic acid) is one of the safest and most effective nutrients, experts say. It may not be the cure for the common cold (though it's thought to help prevent more serious complications), but the benefits of vitamin C may include protection against immune system deficiencies, cardiovascular disease, prenatal health problems, eye disease, and wrinkles.

Vitamin D (cholecalciferol) is essential for promoting calcium absorption in the gut and maintaining adequate serum calcium and phosphate concentrations to enable normal mineralization of bone and prevent hypocalcemic tetany. It is also needed for bone growth and bone remodeling by osteoblasts and osteoclasts. Without sufficient vitamin D, bones can become thin, brittle, or misshapen. Vitamin D sufficiency prevents rickets in children and osteomalacia in adults. Together with calcium, vitamin D also helps protect the elderly from osteoporosis. Vitamin D has other roles in human health, including modulation of neuromuscular and immune function and reduction of inflammation.

Vitamin E describes a family of eight antioxidants, four tocopherols and four tocotrienols. alpha-tocopherol (atocopherol) is the only form of vitamin E that is actively maintained in the human body and is therefore, the form of vitamin E found in the largest quantities in the blood and tissue. Vitamin E, a fat-soluble vitamin, protects vitamin A and essential fatty acids from oxidation in the body cells and prevents breakdown of body tissues.

Vitamin K is needed for blood to properly clot, and for the live to make

blood clotting factors, including factor II (prothrombin), factor VII (proconvertin), factor IX (thromboplastin component), and factor X (Stuart factor). Other clotting factors that depend on vitamin K are protein C, protein S, and protein Z. Deficiency of vitamin K or disturbances of liver function (for example, severe liver failure) may lead to deficiencies of clotting factors and excess bleeding.

Amino Acids: The Foundation of Our Body.

There are 18 different amino acids, or protein types, that are the building blocks for a healthy body. Non-essential amino acids are proteins that the body can synthesize by itself, provided there is enough nitrogen, carbon, hydrogen, and oxygen available. Essential amino acids are proteins supplied by the food you eat. They must be consumed in your diet as the human body either cannot make them or cannot make them in sufficient quantities to meet your body's needs.

Proteins act as enzymes, hormones, and antibodies for your immune system. They maintain fluid balance and keep the levels of acid and alkalinity in check. Proteins also transport substances such as oxygen, vitamins, and minerals to target cells throughout the body. Structural proteins, such as collagen and keratin, are responsible for the formation of bones, teeth, hair, and the outer layer of skin and they help maintain the structure of blood vessels and other tissues.

Enzymes are proteins that facilitate chemical reactions without being changed in the process. Hormones or (chemical messengers) are proteins that travel to one or more specific target tissues or organs, and many have important regulatory functions. Insulin, for example, plays a key role in regulating the amount of glucose in the blood.

The human body also uses protein to manufacture antibodies (giant protein molecules), which combat invading antigens. Antigens are usually foreign substances such as bacteria and viruses that have entered the body and could potentially be harmful. Immunoproteins, also called immunoglobulins or antibodies, defend your body from possible attack from these invaders by binding to the antigens and inactivating them.

If these critical components for a healthy body are not provided as part of a healthy diet, your body will look for other sources for them. This can include the breakdown of your organs, leading to chronic problems such as liver and kidney problems, diabetes, and heart disease.

Moringa Oleifera Leaf Powder Moringa is considered a complete food because it contains all of the essential amino acids required for a healthy body.

DRIED MORINGA LEAF is a nutritional powerhouse and contains all of the following amino acids:

ISOLEUCINE builds proteins and enzymes and it provides ingredients used to create other essential biochemical components in the body, some of which promote energy and stimulate the brain to maintain a state of alertness.

LEUCINE works with isoleucine to build proteins and enzymes which enhance the body's energy and alertness.

LYSINE ensures your body absorbs the right amount of calcium. It also helps form collagen used in bone cartilage and connective tissues. In addition, lysine aids in the production of antibodies, hormones, and enzymes. Recent studies have shown lysine improves the balance of nutrients that reduce viral growth.

METHIONINE primarily supplies sulfur to your body. It is known to prevent hair, skin, and nail problems, while lowering cholesterol levels as it increases the liver's production of lecithin. Methionine reduces liver fat and protects the kidneys, which reduces bladder irritation.

PHENYLALAINE produces the chemical needed to transmit signals between nerve cells and the brain. It can help with concentration and alertness, reduce hunger pains, and improve memory and mood.

THREONINE is an important part of collagen, elastin, and enamel proteins. It assists metabolism and helps prevent fat build-up in the liver while boosting the body's digestive and intestinal tracts.

TRYPTOPHAN supports the immune system, alleviates insomnia, and reduces anxiety, depression, and the symptoms of migraine headaches. It also is beneficial in decreasing the risk of artery and heart spasms as it works with lysine to reduce cholesterol levels.

VALINE is important in promoting a sharp mind, coordinated muscles, and a calm mood.

Non-Essential Amino Acids in Moringa

ALANINE is important for energy in muscle tissue, brain, and central nervous system. It strengthens the immune system by producing antibodies. Alanine also helps in the healthy metabolism of sugars and organic acids in the body.

ARGININE causes the release of the growth hormones considered crucial for optimal muscle growth and tissue repair. It also improves immune responses to bacteria, viruses, and tumor cells while promoting the healing of the body's wounds.

ASPARTIC ACID helps rid the body of ammonia created by cellular waste. When the ammonia enters the circulatory system it can act as a highly toxic substance which can damage the central nervous system. Recent studies have also shown that aspartic acid may decrease fatigue and increase endurance.

CYSTINE functions as an antioxidant and is a powerful aid to the body in protecting against radiation and pollution. It can help slow the aging process, deactivate free radicals, and neutralize toxins. It also helps in protein synthesis and presents cellular change. It is necessary for the formation of new skin cells, which aids in the recovery from burns and surgical operations.

GLUTAMIC ACID is food for the brain. It improves mental capacities, helps speed the healing of ulcers, reduces fatigue, and curbs sugar cravings.

GLYCINE promotes the release of oxygen required in the cell-making process. It is also important in the manufacturing of hormones responsible for a strong immune system. HISTIDINE is used in the treatment of rheumatoid arthritis, allergies, ulcers, and anemia. A lack of histidine may lead to poor hearing.

SERINE is important in storing glucose in the liver and muscles. Its antibodies help strengthen the body's immune system. Plus, it synthesizes fatty acid sheaths around nerve fibers.

PROLINE is extremely important for the proper function of your joints and tendons. It also helps maintain and strengthen heart muscles.

TYROSINE transmits nerve impulses to your brain. It helps overcome depression;

improves memory; increases mental alertness; plus promotes the healthy functioning of the thyroid, adrenal, and pituitary glands.

Here are a few of the many nutritional benefits of Moringa Oleifera, the Miracle Tree:

PROTEIN: Moringa leaves are about 40% protein, with all of the 9 essential amino acids present in various amounts (histidine, isoleucine, leucine, lysine, methionine, phenylalanine, threonine, tryptophan, and valine). Moringa is considered to have the highest protein ratio of any plant so far studied on earth. Moringa has protein quality and quantity similar to soy beans, but there are no reports of Moringa triggered allergies so it can be used for baby nutrition replacing soy. Moringa is not genetically modified or altered by humans.

VITAMINS: Moringa is a vitamin treasure trove. The amounts of betacarotene, Vitamin C and Vitamin E found in Moringa exceed those amounts commonly found in most other plants.

Beta-carotene (pro-vitamin A): Moringa leaves contain more beta-carotene than carrots, about three to five times more, ounce per ounce. There is about 7-8 mg of beta-carotene in 100g (about 3 oz.). The daily recommended value is about 1 mg. The body produces Vitamin A from beta-carotene. It is believed that Vitamin A is the most important vitamin for immune protection against all kinds of infections. It is involved in healing and bone development. Beta-carotene guards against heart disease and can keep harmful lipoproteins containing cholesterol from damaging the heart and coronary arteries. It also helps prevent certain types of cancers and stroke. To provide the best anti-cancer protection, beta-carotene should be present with

Vitamin C and Vitamin E, and Selenium. Moringa has them all.

Vitamin C: Just one ounce of Moringa leaves contains the daily recommended amount of Vitamin C (60 mg). In fact, it is so rich in Vitamin C that, ounce per ounce, it contains 6 – 7 times that found in orange juice. Vitamin C strengthens our immune system and fights infectious diseases including colds and flu.

Vitamin E: Moringa contains large amounts of Vitamin E, at 113 mg per 100 g (about 3 oz.) of the dried leaf powder. The recommended daily intake of Vitamin E is 10 mg. Vitamin E is a potent anti-oxidant that helps prevent premature aging and degenerative diseases including heart disease, arthritis, diabetes and cancer. It also protects the body from pollution, increases stamina and reduces or prevents hot flashes in menopause. It promotes young-looking skin, as well as healing and reducing scar tissue from forming.

Vitamin B1 (Thiamin): Moringa leaves contain high amounts of Vitamin B1 even compared with the best sources already known. It is higher than green peas, black beans (boiled) and corn (boiled). Vitamin B1 is vital for the production of energy in each cell and it plays an essential role in the metabolism of various carbohydrates.

Vitamin B2 (Riboflavin): Moringa leaves compare with broccoli and spinach in Vitamin B2 content. Vitamin B2 is required for the production of energy, proper use of oxygen and the metabolism of amino acids, fats and carbohydrates. It is needed to activate vitamin B6 and assist the adrenal glands. It is important for red blood cell formation, antibody production and growth. And it is required for healthy mucus membranes, skin, and for the absorption of iron and certain vitamins.

Vitamin B3 (Niacin): Moringa leaves and pods contain about 0.5 – 0.8 mg of Vitamin B3 per 100 grams (about 3 ounces). Recommended daily intake is 18 mg. Vitamin B3 is important for energy production and metabolism of protein, fats and carbohydrates. It supports the function of the digestive system and promotes healthy skin and nerves. Vitamins B1, B2 and B3 work synergistically.

Choline: Moringa leaves and pods contain about 423 mg of Choline per 100 g (3 oz.). Diet recommendations call for about 400-550 mg/day. Choline is critical for normal membrane structure and cellular function. It is used by the kidneys to maintain water balance and by the liver for synthesis of various compounds. It is used to produce the important neurotransmitter acetylcholine. It is also vital for the developing fetus and infant.

MINERALS:

Calcium: Ounce per ounce, Moringa leaves contain far higher amounts of calcium than most plants, and 4 times the amount of calcium found in milk. Calcium builds strong bones and teeth and helps prevent osteoporosis.

Iron: Ounce per ounce, Moringa leaves contain over three times the amount of iron found in roast beef, and three times that found in spinach. Iron is necessary for many functions in the body including formation of hemoglobin, brain development and function, regulation of body temperature and muscle activity. Iron is essential for binding oxygen to the blood cells. The central function of iron is oxygen transport and cell respiration.

Potassium: Bananas are an excellent source of potassium but ounce per ounce, Moringa leaves contain three times the potassium of bananas. Potassium is essential for the brain and nerves.

Other minerals that Moringa contains include selenium, zinc, magnesium, phosphorus, copper and sulfur.

ESSENTIAL FATTY ACIDS: Moringa oleifera leaves and seeds contain beneficial essential fatty acids (EFA's). Moringa seeds contain between 30-42% oil, with 13% saturated fats and 82% unsaturated fatty acids. Oleifera is the Latin term for "oil containing." About 73% of the Moringa oil is oleic acid, while in most beneficial plant oils, oleic acid only contributes up to 40%. Olive oil is about 75% oleic acid, and sunflower is about 20%. Oleic acid is linked to lower rates of cardiovascular disease, neurological disease, artherosclerosis, infections, and certain types of cancer, and it helps to regulate blood glucose levels.

OTHER NUTRIENTS FOUND IN MORINGA:

CHLOROPHYLL: Moringa is one of the few foods that contain chlorophyll together with so many other nutrients. Chlorophyll is often referred to as the 'blood of plants." Studies have shown that it supports liver function and detoxification of the body.

BETA-SITOSTEROL: Beta-sitosterol is a specific plant sterol which has been shown to reduce blood cholesterol levels and also improve other blood lipid levels, bringing them to a more normal range. Plant sterols like beta-sitosterol are also proven to be very beneficial in preventing and treating prostate enlargement due to aging, and have been found to reduce the growth of prostate and colon cancer cells. Beta-sitosterol also boosts the immune system, has anti-inflammatory properties, helps normalize blood sugar, supports the pancreas, helps to heal ulcers and can alleviate cramps.

ZEATIN: Biochemical analysis has revealed that the Moringa leaves and leaf powder contain unusually high amounts of plant hormones named cytokinins, such as zeatin and the related dihyrozeatin. Scientists have found zeatin in very low concentrations in plants, with zeatin concentrations varying between .00002 mcg/g material to .02 mcg/g. The zeatin concentration in Moringa leaves gathered from various parts of the world was found to be very high, between 5 mcg and 200 mcg/g material, or thousands of times more concentrated than most plants studied so far.

Cytokinins function as plant hormones, which are naturally occurring growth promoters and factors that delay the process of aging in many plants. In cultured human cells, cytokinins have proven to delay biochemical modifications associated with aging. Zeatin has potent antioxidant properties, and has been shown to protect the skin and increase the activity of known antioxidant enzymes that naturally fight aging. It has also been shown to protect animals against neuronal toxicity induced by age specific factors, and in the laboratory setting, to inhibit cancer cell growth and induce their differentiation back into normal cells.

LUTEIN: Moringa has extraordinary amounts of lutein. 100 g of leaves contain more than 70 mg, while the recommended daily amount for the best protective antioxidant activity is 5 – 20 mg for an adult. Lutein promotes healthy eyes by reducing the risk of macular degeneration.

CAFFEOYLQUINIC ACIDS: Moringa leaves contain 0.5 – 1% caffeoylquinic acids, coming very close to the content that makes artichokes famous. Caffeoylquinic acids are antioxidants considered to be choleretic (bile increasing which helps to digest dietary fats), hepatoprotective (effective against hepatitis and other liver diseases), cholesterol-reducing, and diuretic.

NOTE: Complex mixtures of naturally occurring antioxidants from plants are the most effective and beneficial protectors against oxidation and aging. Moringa contains many other antioxidants including alpha carotene, xanthins, kaempferol, quercetin, and rutin. **(Sandra Toliver)**

This is God's Superfood that's ready, willing and able to meet your health and wellness needs in today's society. The most nutritious tree ever discovered and contains no fillers, additives, preservatives, etc... just 100% Superior Grade Moringa Oleifera.

4

The Leaves of the Tree

"And the leaves of the tree were for the healing of the nations." Rev. 22:2c

There is a tree which has healing in its leaves according to the word of God. I believe that this is a two-fold message that speaks to us today as well as a future word about a particular tree. If you will notice it does not say that **"the leaves of the trees**—but **the leaves of the tree."** Meaning that it's only a particular tree or one tree that has leaves which has healing properties in it. The scriptures say, *"And he shewed me a pure river of water of life, clear as crystal, proceeding out of the throne of God and of the Lamb. In the midst of the street of it, and on either side of the river, was there the tree of life, which bare twelve manner of fruits, and yielded her fruit every month:* **and the leaves of the tree were for the healing of the nations."** *Revelation 22:1-2*

Spiritually speaking this scripture tells

us about a time when the nations or the redeemed shall be gathered out of every nation according to Revelation 21:24 which states *"And the nations of them which are saved shall walk in the light of it: and the kings of the earth do bring their glory and honour into it."* Also the book of Ezekiel 47:12 tells us about the leaves of a tree which will be used for healing as it states, *"And by the river upon the bank thereof, on this side and on that side, shall grow all trees for meat, whose leaf shall not fade, neither shall the fruit thereof be consumed: it shall bring forth new fruit according to his months, because their waters they issued out of the sanctuary: and the fruit thereof shall be for meat, and **the leaf thereof for medicine.**"*

The nations that do bring their glory in the new Jerusalem will have access to this tree and will need it not to abstain from sickness or disease but to keep their body in health just as Adam had to eat to keep his body in health and:

- Full of life

- Vibrant

- Dynamic

- Healthy

- Flourishing

- Thriving

- Totally Alive

- Robust

- Nothing Missing

- Nothing Lacking

- Whole

- Top Form

- Full of Strength

- Sustained

- And Sound…

If you will notice also this tree as stated

according to Ezekiel will have some fruit on it but the medicine or healing will not be in the fruit but in the leaves. They will have to eat the leaves and when they eat them it will cause a vibrancy of health and sustainability of their body as a result of the nutrients within. These leaves will possess a quality of life that will be like eating leaves of life.

The natural aspect of the leaves of the tree for today has a different connotation because today we are dealing with sickness and diseases. The leaves of the tree for the healing of the nation today will be used exactly as stated—for healing. You can go through every list of Superfoods that's out today and there are many that God created that are excellent for our bodies. I've always stated that there are only two reasons or uses for medicine:

1. For emergencies such as someone in a car accident or someone that needs an immediate surge for pain-

killer or to halt an immediate medical need.

2. God does not want you to die from a sickness or disease that can be halted or symptoms that can be eased by the use of medication. It's not God's first choice but for those that don't have faith for divine healing or refuses to use God's leaves, plants, herbs for health restoration then medicine it is. Stay alive at all cost but believe God for healing and or use his remedy for health and restoration. Get off medicine as quick as you can.

God's Superfood is his remedy to prevent sickness and disease or to restore you back to health and wellness. There is no other Superfood on the planet that can compare with **the leaves of Moringa Oleifera.**

5

The Power of Moringa Powder

As great as the leaves are most people prefer to use the Moringa powder instead of the leaves.

The powder is more preferred than the leaves because as potent as the leaves are we've found that the powder converted from the Moringa leaves gives it more potency than the leaves themselves. When the leaves are dried and then changed into Moringa powder the nutritional content increases by over 10 times. So the nutritional value of the powder is far more superior to the nutritional value of the leaves yet the powder converted maintains the potency:

- 3 times the Potassium in bananas.

- 7 times the Vitamin-C as in oranges.

- 25 times the Iron in spinach.

- 4 times the Calcium in milk.

- 4 times the Vitamin A in Carrots.

- 20 times more Vitamin E than Tofu.

- 2 times more Protein than Eggs.

- 10 times more Vitamin E than Nuts.

- 9 times the protein of yogurt.

When you take a single tablespoon of the Moringa powder you are receiving the daily recommended allowance of nutritional value. The benefits of using Moringa are so astronomical that we don't have enough space to list all the things that Moringa does. We suggest that you start out with a single teaspoon of the Moringa powder and you can eventually increase it after 90 days if you desire or remain at a single teaspoon.

The Moringa powder is easily used and a teaspoon can be added to a variety of things such as:

- Moringa in **a bottle of water.**

- Moringa in **smoothie.**

- Moringa in **oatmeal.**

- Moringa in **rice.**

- Moringa in **yogurt.**

- Moringa in **juices.**

- Moringa in **salads.**

- Moringa in **soups.**

- Moringa in **stews.**

- Moringa in **coffee.**

- Moringa in **Guacamole**

- Moringa can be added to just about anything.

The one thing to remember when cooking with Moringa is to put it in at the conclusion of your meal cooking. The last 5 to 10 minutes is good so that the excess heat will not destroy some of the vitamins and enzymes of the Moringa powder or leaves. The powder is an easy method to take Moringa and the taste is sort of like kale, spinach, or a natural leafy taste.

The Moringa powder is very high in protein which helps to support the growth and maintenance of muscle mass.

The Moringa powder has been used for thousands of years for its medicinal properties and health benefits.

The Moringa powder is a plant free of chemicals and that is comprised of 90+ Nutrients, 46 + Antioxidants, 36 AntiInflammatory Compounds, 18 + Amino Acids and 8 Essential Amino Acids—the ones your body cannot survive without but cannot manufacture on its own.

The Moringa powder is considered a superfood that builds up your immune system and fights off free radicals.

The Moringa powder removes toxins from your body and detoxifies your body as well as removes parasites from your body.

The Moringa powder contains both antimicrobial and antibacterial properties.

The Moringa powder contains phytonutrients like zeatin, quercetin, beta-sistosterol, caffeeoylquinic acid and kaempferol.

The Moringa powder reduces the inflammation in the body without side effects.

The Moringa powder protects the liver and kidneys as a result of the minerals that are derived from this plant.

The Moringa powder has antibacterial, antifungal, antimicrobial, properties that can help combat infections and get or keep you on the road to health and wellness.

The Moringa powder keeps the body balance because the body now has the essential nutrients needed to protect it and now your body works with you instead of against you.

The Moringa powder strengthens your immune system or defense system and a strong immune system means a strong physical body.

The Moringa powder makes your body more alkaline and when your body is more alkaline then you're on the path to health and wellness.

We encourage you in the conclusion of this book Moringa Oleifera—The Tree of Life to realize that God has not left man alone to fight sickness. God is good and in his goodness he has given us three things to combat sickness and disease.

1. **Spiritual gifts** or **gifts of the Holy Spirit** of healings, working of miracles and faith so that the people

of God will have the advantage over sickness and diseases. 1 Corinthians 12

2. As saints of the Most High God if there is any sick among us we can also *"call for the elders of the church; and let them pray over him, anointing him with oil in the name of the Lord: And the prayer of faith shall save the sick, and the Lord will raise him up; and if he hath committed sins, they shall be forgiven him" James 5:14-15*

3. Lastly, the herbs of the fields and the leaves of the tree for there is a plant for every illness known to man. And Moringa Oleifera is the most powerful Superfood ever discovered to date.

You have within your reach a God given plant that can give you your life back and help you to live a better quality of life. Do you want it? Will you accept it? I wonder, but time and action will tell!

6

Make the Rest of Your Life
The Best of Your Life

Sickness and disease is your enemy and throughout the word of God you see Jesus going about eradicating sickness and disease from the life of man. The scripture says, *"How God anointed Jesus of Nazareth with the Holy Ghost and with power: who went about **doing good**, and **healing all** that were oppressed of the devil; for God was with him." Acts 10:38*

It's hard to have a good life with sickness and disease ravaging your body. Maybe in the past you did not know that sickness and disease were an enemy and felt like you were doomed to this fate. But we want to let you know that God wants you to make the rest of your life the best of your life. God sent Jesus to do 3 things:

1. To reconcile man back to God through repentance unto salvation. 2 Corinthians 5:14-19, Romans 10:8-

13, Mark 1:15, Mark 2:17

2. To deliver mankind from the curse of sickness and disease. Isaiah 53, 1 Peter 2:24, Acts 10:38, Matthew 8:16, Matthew 12:15, Mark 2:1-12,

3. To deliver mankind from the curse of poverty. 3 John 2, Philippians 4:19, Psalms 23:1, 2 Corinthians 9:8, Romans 8:32

We see here as in many other scriptures that Jesus came to set mankind free in spirit, soul and body. This is total life prosperity and if one of these is missing then life is not dispensing to you all that you can have or be. However, in this book our focus is on your physical health so it's the will of God that you are in good health in order for you to truly enjoy life.

There were many occasions where Jesus went about healing people to get rid of their sickness with a touch and command from the master. This is called divine healing or healing without the aid of medicine or natural herbs of any kind. The scripture says, "*32 And at even, when the sun did set, they brought unto him all that were diseased, and them that were possessed with devils.*

33 And all the city was gathered together at the door.

34 And he healed many that were sick of divers diseases, and cast out many devils; and suffered not the devils to speak, because they knew him." Mark 1:32-34

Divine healing is always God's first and best method for many reasons:

1. *It brings glory and honor to God alone.*

2. *It's doesn't cost mankind anything.*

3. *It can draw mankind closer to God and show them the reality of God.*

So I admonish you to seek God for your healing and he's faithful that promised. But also remember that sickness is an enemy and that God doesn't want it attached to your body in any form or fashion. If you haven't been healed by the power of God then know that God has created the herbs of the field for healing and restoration. We've seen many cases where the leaves of the Moringa tree have restored sick bodies as well as been used for the prevention of sickness and disease.

You have to learn to take personal responsibility for your health and wellness. Don't sick back and wait on anyone to do for you what you can do for yourself.

- Stop feeling sorry for yourself and your condition.

- Stop having a pity party and rise up.

- Stop been passive about your health.

- Become proactive about your health.

- Take charge of your own health and do something to get better.

- Arise from your position of do nothing and do something for health and wellness.

From a natural perspective God has given the human race a plant that can restore their health. This plant is full of everything your body needs for health and wellness. This plant is able to help fight off inflammation which is a major indicator for sickness and disease.

Inflammation inputs a major component towards sickness and disease in your body and can cause chronic inflammation overtime. When chronic inflammation continues for a long time then cell damages occur and lead to a variety of sickness and diseases. Some of the sickness and diseases cause by inflammation are:

- Arthritis

- Rheumatism

- Asthma

- Dermatitis

- Sarcoidosis

- Lupus

- Tuberculosis

- Sinusitis

- Cancer

- Ulcerative Colitis

- Crohn's Disease

- Inflammatory Bowel Disease

- Multiple Sclerosis

- Heart attacks

- Most Strokes

- Peripheral Artery Disease

- Vascular Dementia

- Multiple Sclerosis

- Diabetes

- Atherosclerosis

- Periodontitis

- Hay fever

- Heart disease,

- And much more…

Moringa Oleifera is an anti-inflammatory food that helps with inflammatory conditions due to its 36 anti-inflammatory compounds within. When inflammation is lessen in your body then your body can fight off more sickness and diseases. There is no other food on the market today that can fight inflammation better than Moringa Oleifera. With all the antioxidants and amino acids within this tree it's truly a modern day tree of life.

What would people do today if God told them that there was a tree of life located in a certain location and the leaves of that tree could cause health and wellness in your body?

The leaves of this tree could prevent sickness and diseases from entering your body.

The leaves of this tree could build up your immune system and when your system is strong then your body is strong and vibrant and able to resist diseases.

The leaves of this tree could fight off free radicals and help deter cancer.

The leaves of this tree could remove toxins from your body as well as detoxify your body.

The leaves of this tree could remove parasites from your body which causes much sickness and diseases.

The leaves of this tree have no side effects because it's truly all natural.

The leaves of this tree is giving people hope and when hope is present then people have expectation of a better life.

The leaves of this tree contain antimicrobial properties.

The leaves of this tree provide the essential nutrients for a health liver and kidneys.

The leaves of this tree can fight off infections because of the antibacterial properties within.

The leaves of this tree keep your body balance and a balanced body is a healthy body.

The leaves of this tree make your body alkaline and give it a pH greater than 7.

Well there is such a tree and the leaves of the tree are for healing and restoration and it's our modern day tree of life called Moringa Oleifera.

- Why should you die before your time?

- Why should you die when others are living?

- Why should you throw in the towel just because you have been diagnosed with cancer?

- You can live and declare the works of the Lord

- You can take your life back.

- You can have life and have it more abundantly.

- You can triumph over sickness and disease.

- You can get your life back.

- You can throw the towel back and refuse to accept the diagnosis.

- You can accept God's Superfood as an aid, help and service for mankind.

- You can believe that God does not want you to die of sickness and disease but become proactive.

You can live the rest of your life the best of your life by partaking of this modern day tree of life called Moringa Oleifera. Life is a blessing but you must also fight for your life and not give in to the wiles of the devil that comes to steal, kill and destroy. John 10:10

Become more proactive and learn what you need to know not only for your life but for your family, your friends, your neighbors and as many people as you can reach. Take action and do it now, if you do you will indeed make the rest of your life the best of your life by partaking of Moringa Oleifera — The Tree of Life.

See Our List of Other Books About Moringa:

1. The Greatest Plant on the Planet
2. Moringa Over Medicine
3. The Beelzebub Letters (A serious of 5 books)
4. The Breakthrough Oil That's Changing Lives –Moringa Oleifra

Eden Wellness Moringa
123 N. Center Street
Goldsboro, NC 27530
www.edenwellnessmoringa.com
edenwellness@yahoo.com

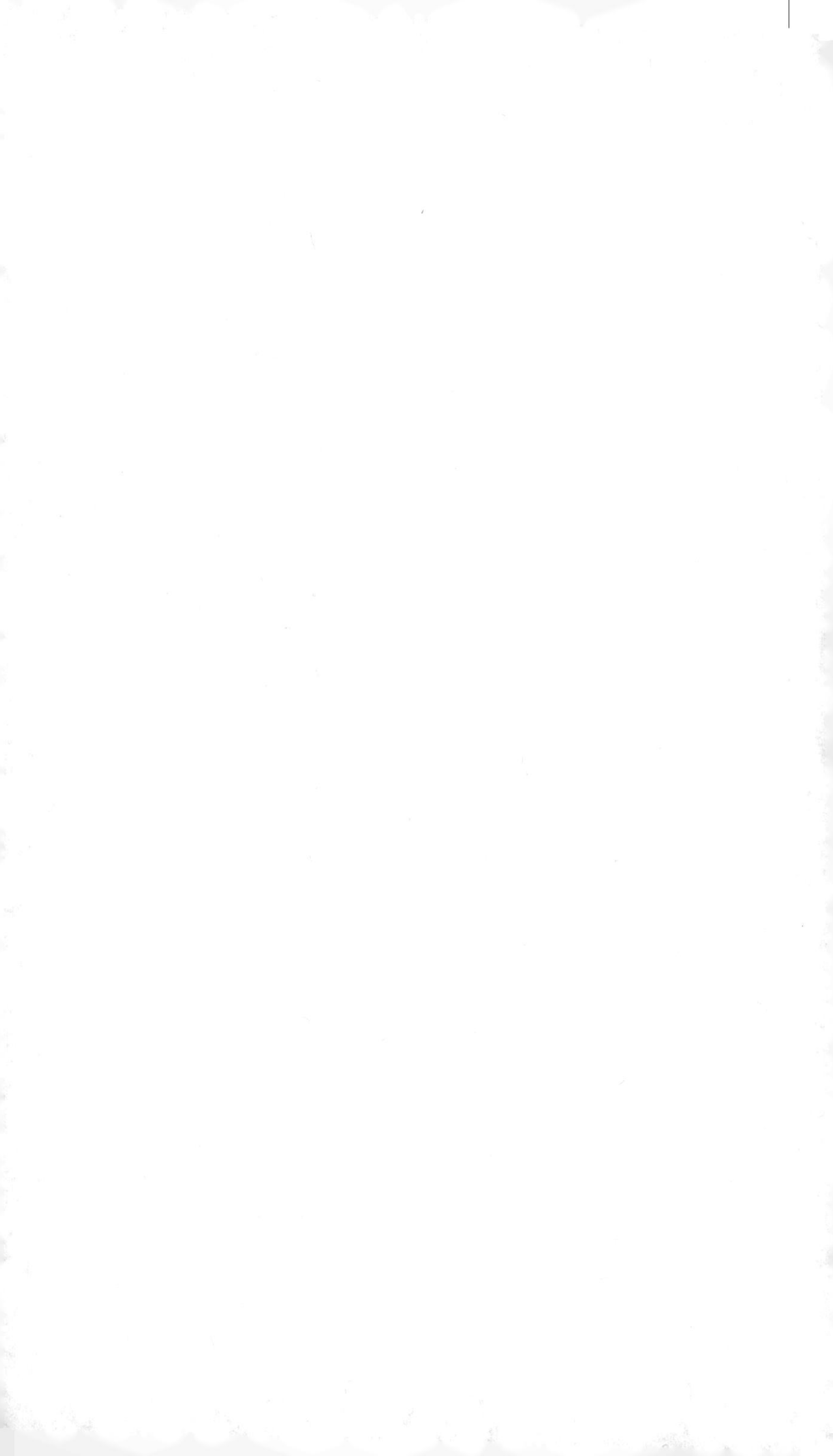